Brain Injury Survivor's Prayer

God,

I come before You as one whose injury
Cannot be seen by your other children.

While others see me, they know not that
My wounds are invisible.

I come before you as a
Brain injury survivor.

You alone know the depth of my pain,
Of my despair, of my confusion, of my aloneness,
And of my overwhelming loss of self.

Humbly, I ask of You...

When exhaustion strikes, please
Grant me the strength I need to continue.

When others leave my life, help me to
Remember that You are always there with me.

When unsteadiness causes me to stumble,
Please take my hand and lead me safely forward.

When my memory so often fails me,
Help me to never forget what is really important.

God, so many of your children walk daily with
Challenges that dwarf my own.

By understanding this, I can see my own
Life in a better perspective.

Help me for today to accept my fate in this life
Knowing that if I trust in you,
All will be well.

Amen.

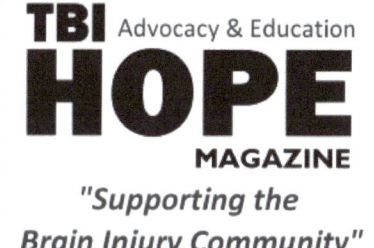

TBI Advocacy & Education
HOPE
MAGAZINE

*"Supporting the
Brain Injury Community"*

Welcome

TBI HOPE MAGAZINE

Serving All Impacted by Brain Injury

June 2017

Publisher
David A. Grant

Editor
Sarah Grant

Contributing Writers
Amiee Duffy
Aislinn Fallon
Debra Gorman
Kelly Lang
Norma Myers
Jayden Pollack
Lisa Rainaud
Sherry White

Amazing Cartoonist
Patrick Brigham

FREE subscriptions at
www.TBIHopeMagazine.com

Welcome to the June 2017 issue of TBI HOPE Magazine!

During a recent conversation with my wife Sarah, we spoke about the types of articles which have made TBI HOPE Magazine so popular within the brain injury community.

Beginning with our first issue back in 2015, we made the decision not to candy-coat the true reality of life after brain injury. We did this mindful of our readers. If every story we published was a *happily ever after* story, we would be rendering a huge disservice to you.

We chose to show examples of life after brain injury as it really is: raw, often difficult, but most of all, achievable. The courage and perseverance of our contributing writers continues to amaze me.

The fact that these brave souls are willing to be transparent and tell the world of their struggles, hardships and victories is a reminder that courage is indeed found in unlikely places.

It is our hope that you enjoy this issue of TBI HOPE Magazine for what it is – a reflection of the lives of some pretty amazing people.

Peace,

David A. Grant
Publisher

Contents

What's Inside

June 2017

Brain Injury Does Not Discriminate Based on Age, Gender, or Nationality

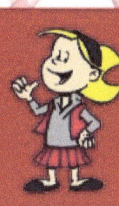

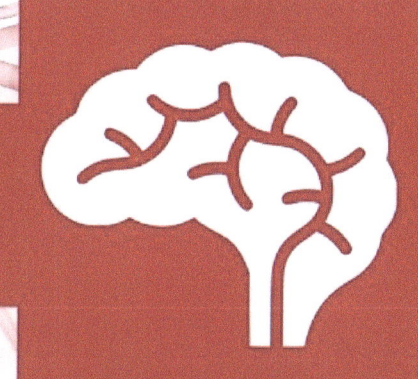

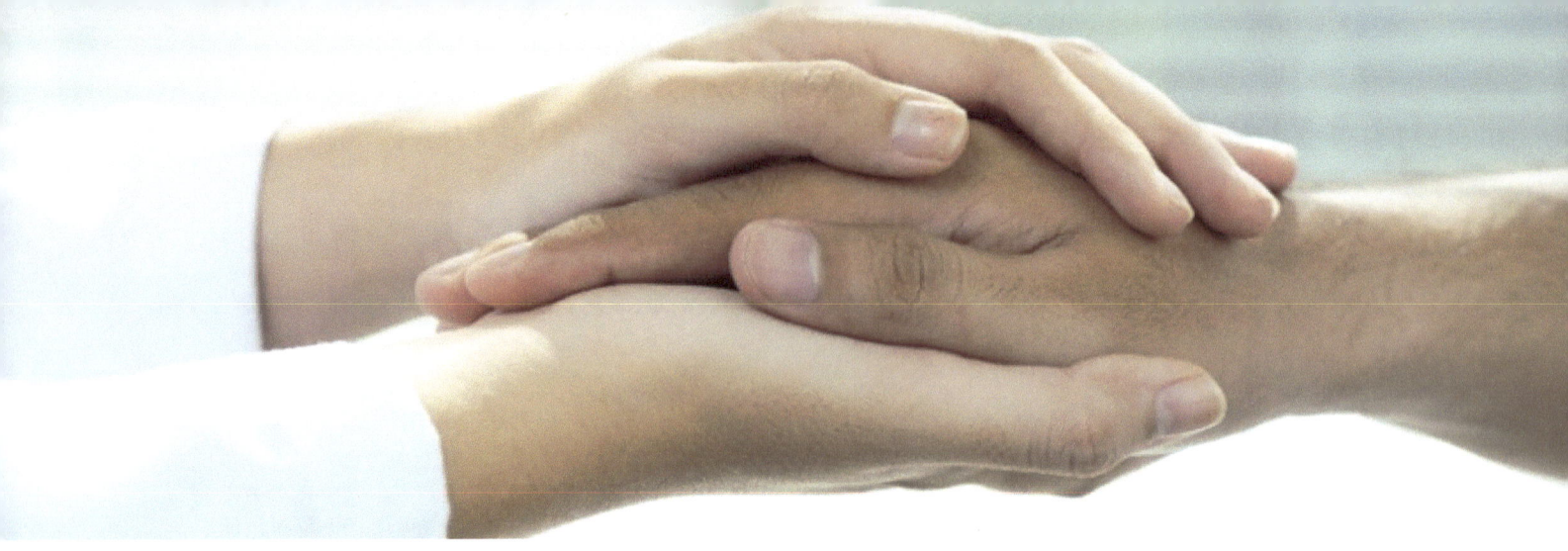

A Matter of Pride

By Debra Gorman

At first, I didn't think I could bear it since it was the most difficult thing I ever had to accept. Having so recently achieved some personal and career goals, I didn't know how to be so different. I went from (by outward appearance) being "together" and successful, to being "disabled" in the blink of an eye.

My brain hemorrhage (an inoperable brainstem cavernous angioma, plus a stroke) happened nearly five years ago. It has been quite a journey, and I have come a long way. In fact, I'm amazed when I look back over the last five years. I worked very hard for improvement that didn't come. I struggled mightily to accept my new reality. I couldn't imagine a life of not "normal." I was heartbroken for a long time. Strangely, I have discovered this new "normal" to be a gift—of sorts. It has stretched me and taught me things I might never have known about myself. For example, I am a person of courage. I don't think I knew that before. I certainly hadn't been tested to this degree. Everyone suffers in this life. Allowing that suffering to mold and shape us into a person with greater compassion, vulnerability and wisdom is a choice, one that can make all the difference.

This white, middle-class woman has now had an inside look at being a "minority" and I am humbled. I never dreamed this would be my life. Once, my neurosurgeon talked to my husband as if I was not in the room. I have been ignored in public places and glanced away from. Mostly, people stare. I imagine they are thinking, "What's wrong with her? Is she drunk? Is she mentally retarded? Hmmm, what's her deal?"

I have also seen the best of humanity. People sometimes go out of their way to help me, and not in a condescending way. Those people are often acquainted with disability or pain in some personal way. They have empathy. They do not back away due to their own discomfort. They move toward me, engage me, and ask how they might support me. I appreciate those people.

I find I have more confidence than ever before, which doesn't make sense on the face of it. I have always had my share of insecurities. I believe that there are no accidents in life. To me, that means that God cares about me so much that he allowed my circumstances knowing I would become better acquainted with him and his grace.

Although my pride took a terrific hit when "disabled" became my new label, I know that pride is a trait to subjugate. I am not my disability, but neither was I my career success. I am a child of God, created in his image. He doesn't love me any greater than he loves someone else, but he loves me a lot. He gives me value and significance; that is what I try to embrace. The challenges put in my path are meant to help me become a better representative of his love.

It has not been an easy process. When I received a handicap parking tag soon after my brain injury, I refused to use it. I would rather navigate long and difficult terrain on foot than succumb to an admission of "handicapped." It only took one Midwest January to get over that bit of pride. I had often imagined myself as an elderly woman; a brain hemorrhage was never part of the plan. I saw myself in my seventies and eighties as a feisty old lady who still backpacked and spent an abundant amount of time in nature.

I was strong and wiry, doing things that old ladies probably shouldn't do. These days my husband and I try to find and capitalize on activities we can still enjoy together. I have always been independent. That can-do attitude has served me well. I look for deeper meaning in life's circumstances and endeavor to be taught and positively changed by the challenges set before me.

> **"**
>
> **When I received a handicap parking tag soon after my brain injury, I refused to use it.**
>
> **"**

It strengthens me physically and mentally to do for myself as much as possible, even if doing so looks nothing like it would have in the past. It usually takes twice as long and is half as good.

I don't think people always understand I am physically - not mentally - compromised. As a nurse, I had been given immediate responsibility and authority. I mourned and had to overcome my feelings of resentment when I wasn't trusted with simple things in my present state. It's that pride thing again.

My husband and I had been married only six wonderful years when I had this devastating brain hemorrhage. I'm sure this journey has not been easy for him, but that's his story and I'll let him tell it when he's ready.

Hope is being able to see that there is light despite all of the darkness.

~Desmond Tutu

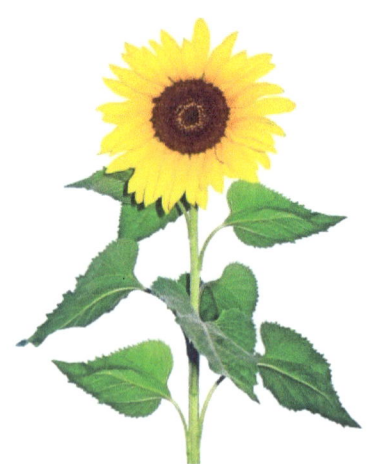

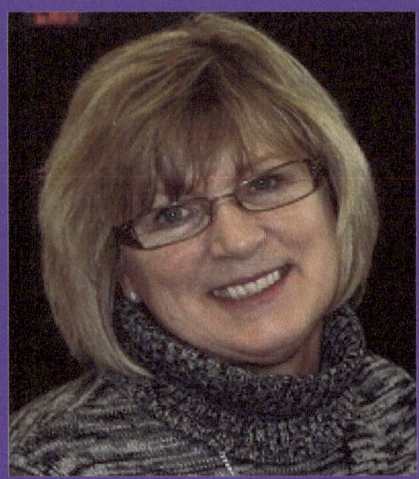

Meet Debra Gorman

Debra Gorman survived a brain hemorrhage from a brain stem cavernous angioma (a congenital condition), August 2011, at fifty-six years old. She had married the love of her life only six years before her injury.

Three months after the first brain bleed she experienced a subdural hematoma, resulting in a craniotomy.

She nearly died several times during those two episodes and family members arrived from all over the country to possibly say goodbye.

Because she survived, she is convinced her life has a new, more focused, purpose. She is grateful to be living, and for the abilities she has retained.

She writes a blog entitled Graceful Journey, which she began well before the brain injury, but since then, has focused more on the commonality of suffering.

www.debralynn48.wordpress.com

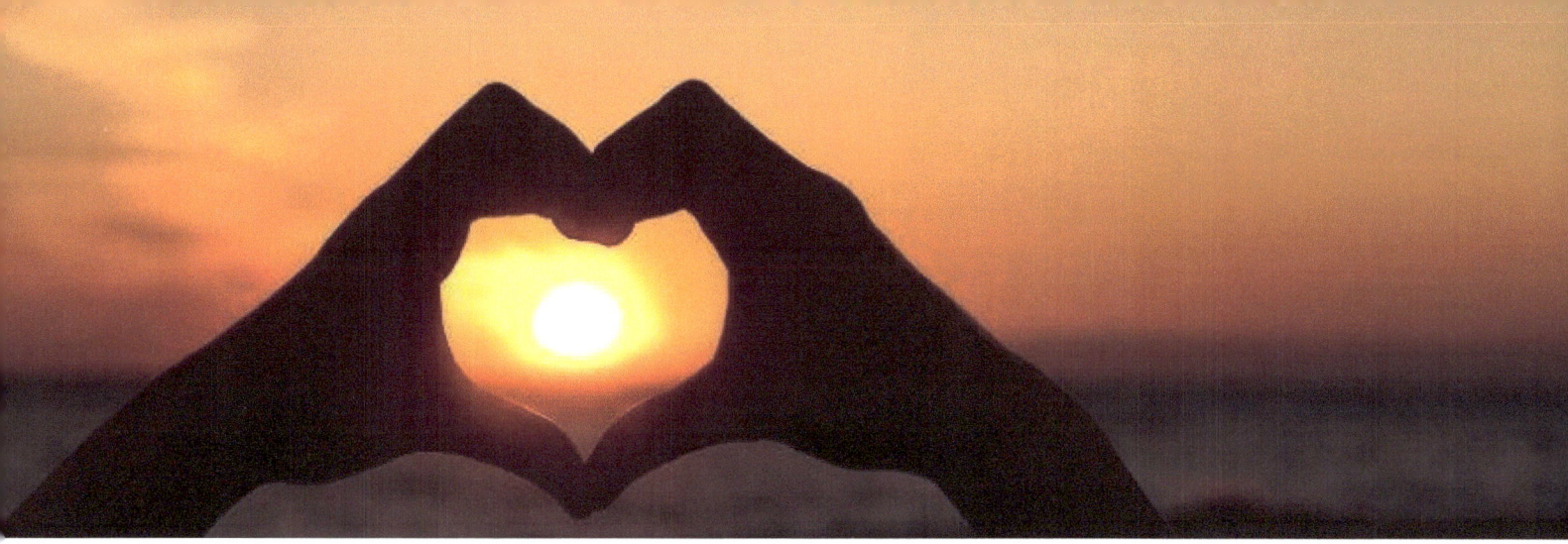

Thankful to be Alive
By Sherry White

My name is Sherry White and I am 51 years old. My husband, granddaughter and I live in Old Saybrook, Connecticut. I work part-time as a Recreation Assistant at a nursing home.

I have had horses all my life. They involved a lot of time and hard labor. As the years passed caring daily for horses, it had taken a toll on my back. Constantly lifting hay and saddles, and bags of grain, my back had finally given out. After several cortisone injections and physical therapy, my doctor discovered through an MRI, a bulging disc in my lower spine and recommended a Laminectomy.

My doctor scheduled an outpatient surgery but I declined. I told him that I preferred to stay overnight because my granddaughter was only two year's old and that I would not be able to care for her right after surgery. Thank God I asked to stay overnight or I wouldn't be writing my story right now.

On December 4th, 2009 at approximately 6:00 am, I was wheeled into the operating room at Middlesex Hospital, in Middletown, Connecticut. After surgery and in the recovery room, I discovered I couldn't move my legs; I was paralyzed from the waist down. After screaming for the doctor, I was once again wheeled back into the same operating room. The paralysis was corrected and I was transferred up to a private room.

My parents came that night to visit. My mother states that I was complaining of a bad headache, and she didn't think the nurses should have gotten me out of bed to use the bathroom so early after the surgery. I have no memory of this. In the early morning, I was found lethargic by my nurse and it was determined that I had a bleed in my brain. I needed to be transferred immediately to a trauma hospital. The closest was Yale New-Haven Hospital, about forty-five minutes away by ambulance. I was transferred by LifeStar, a medical helicopter.

On arrival, I was met by Dr. Joseph Piepmeir, Chief of Neurosurgery, who performed an emergency craniotomy. My forehead was drilled to relieve the pressure building up in my brain and I was transferred up to ICU.

On December 11th, a week later, I was bleeding for the SECOND time in my brain. Back to the operating room for another craniotomy. After surgery, I was returned back up to the ICU floor. I don't have any memory of this. I had been unconscious since leaving Middlesex Hospital.

On December 17th, a week later, I was bleeding again for the THIRD time in my brain. I was taken back to the operating room for another craniotomy. This time, Dr. Piepmeir left out the bone flap in the back of my head, just in case he needed to get back in again saving precious time.

After a few weeks and no more bleeding, I was finally starting to heal. I was only able to hear at this point, but I still did not know what had happened. I started having hallucinations. I thought I had been kidnapped and someone stole Hallie, my grand-daughter. I was totally petrified and scared.

Anytime the nurse gave me pills, I would wait for them to leave and spit them out. I remember demanding my cell phone from my husband. Not able to see, I dialed 911. I told the operator that I had been kidnapped and to please send the police. My behavior at this point was intolerable to both the doctors/nurses and to my family. I was put into a strait jacket and wrist restraints. Now I really thought I was kidnapped, and I needed to escape!

When I was being fed by a nurse, she happened to leave a butter knife on my bed. With my wrists underneath, I was able to grab the butter knife. Late at night, I would try to use the knife to cut off my wrist restraints. I still have nightmares to this day. I had to quit my job as Director of Lymes Senior Center, which I loved. I was now disabled and on disability.

By looking at me you can't tell I am a TBI survivor (three TBI's, actually) which could be good or bad.

Now I really thought I was kidnapped, and I needed to escape!

Good that I look normal, and bad that family and friends don't understand why I have bad days. I know other TBI survivors can relate. My husband didn't like the new me and filed for divorce. He wanted to sue the doctor for wasting his time visiting me in the hospital.

Today, I am very thankful and blessed that I am alive. I don't get angry or upset easily. Life is too short. I have remarried to a great guy who accepts me the way I am. I have also adopted Hallie (that's another story for later).

I see a Psychiatrist for PTSD. I get flashbacks when hearing or smelling anything medically related.

When I get headaches, I panic thinking I am having another brain bleed. If I see a ball flying in the air, I duck for fear the ball will hit me in the head where it is extremely sensitive, like a soft spot. The bone flap was never replaced.

Dr. Piepmeir has told me that he has never known anyone having three craniotomies, nor has he ever performed three craniotomies himself. So, as I count my blessings to three: Ready, Set, Go... Thank you, God!

Meet Sherry White

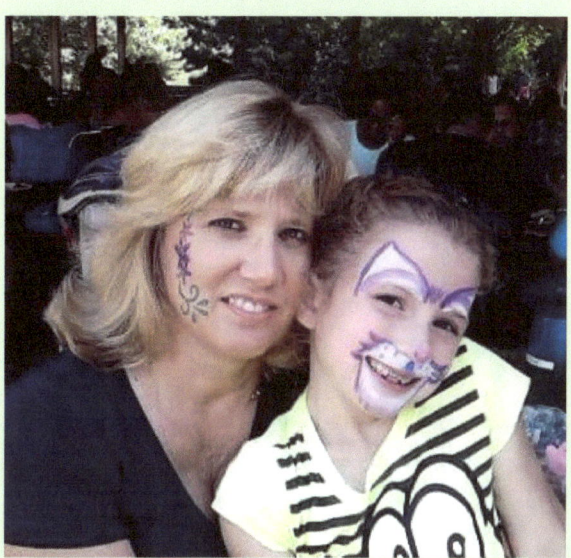

Sherry White is from Connecticut and is a survivor of multiple brain injuries. She is a devoted wife and grandmother. Her first book, 'Coming Out of Darkness,' will be available later this year on Amazon. Sherry hopes that by sharing her own story, others can find hope and realize that they are no longer alone in their struggles.

Living With Hope

By Patrick Brigham

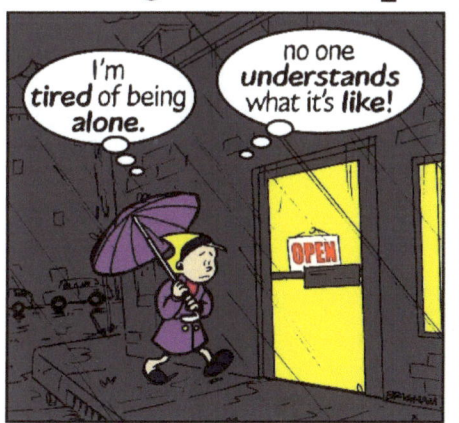
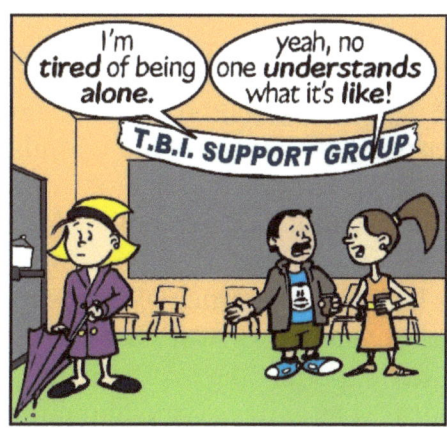
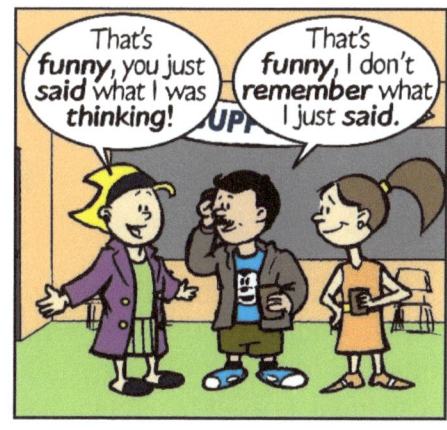

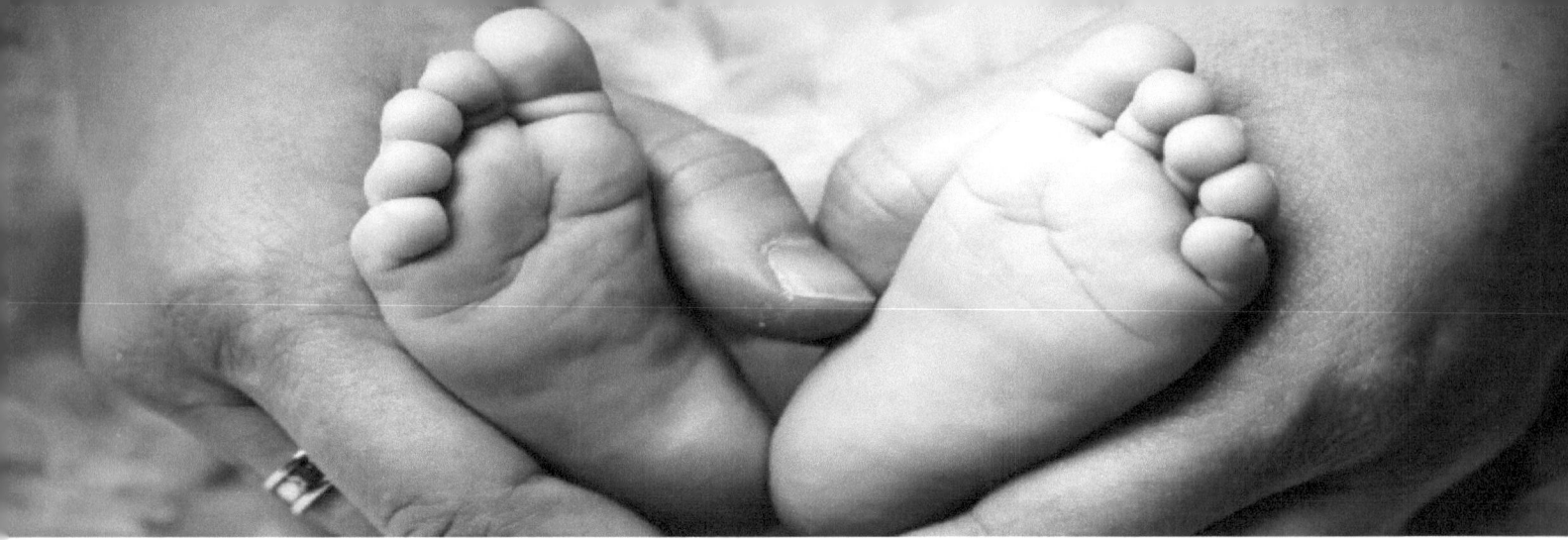

The Birth of Joy

By Kelly Lang

I was starting to emerge from the fog of newborn days and I had recovered some sleep during the past few days. I was happy to be at home with this new bundle of life. She was perfect. I regained enough energy and settled into somewhat of a routine; well, as much of a routine as you can with a newborn baby.

The only sound I remember is Mike, my husband, telling me that until this new baby of ours was born, he had not experienced joy in the past six-and-a-half years. It was the time of day between the afternoon and early evening; the sun was still out but had begun to dip lower in the sky. We were in the kitchen while I was trying to prepare dinner and he was holding our youngest daughter, Anya, as she lay sleeping contently in his arms. She was small but looked especially so in his arms. Early evening in our house is usually a flurry of activity especially since bringing a newborn into the mix. We now had three girls and the outside sounds of laughter, tears, music, fighting, and/or homework were not in my periphery.

My first thought after hearing this confession was WOW! How did I not know this? We had shared a tragedy and yet I had no idea that the depth of his pain reached so far. Our lives had seemed more settled than they previously were. It was the spring of 2008, and our two girls were aged 9 and 11. We had been living in our suburban home in a nice neighborhood and his job was stable after many years of instability in the job markets, due to the aftermath of September 11.

Our beautiful and very different girls had friends, participated in extracurricular activities, and appeared to be well-adjusted given the previous tragedy. They were both so ecstatic to learn we would be adding another child to our mix, especially after experiencing my miscarriage the previous year. Hannah, the oldest and a worrier by nature, had been tentatively excited about this new baby, but cautious due to the previous year's miscarriage which threw her off kilter. Although neither one of them would admit it, I think they were both relieved to learn that their new sibling was a girl. In fact, upon hearing the news, Hannah burst into tears of happiness.

So, how did I not notice the depths of Mike's pain? Was I that self-centered, worrying too much about Olivia's situation and my own, oblivious to my husband's feelings?

The year 2001 started off so bright and full of promise. I was a stay at home mom to two beautiful girls and we were living in a nice neighborhood. Our home was small, and since the real estate market was booming we thought it might be the time to upgrade, although we had only been living in our home for a little over two years. We decided we would build a bigger home just a few miles from our current address. We moved into our new home in November 2001.

A week after our move, while still trying to unpack and organize a house full of furniture, clothing, toys, books, and the million other things we had accumulated over the past eight years of married life, our world started to crumble block by block, each appearing to be worse than the previous. First, Olivia,

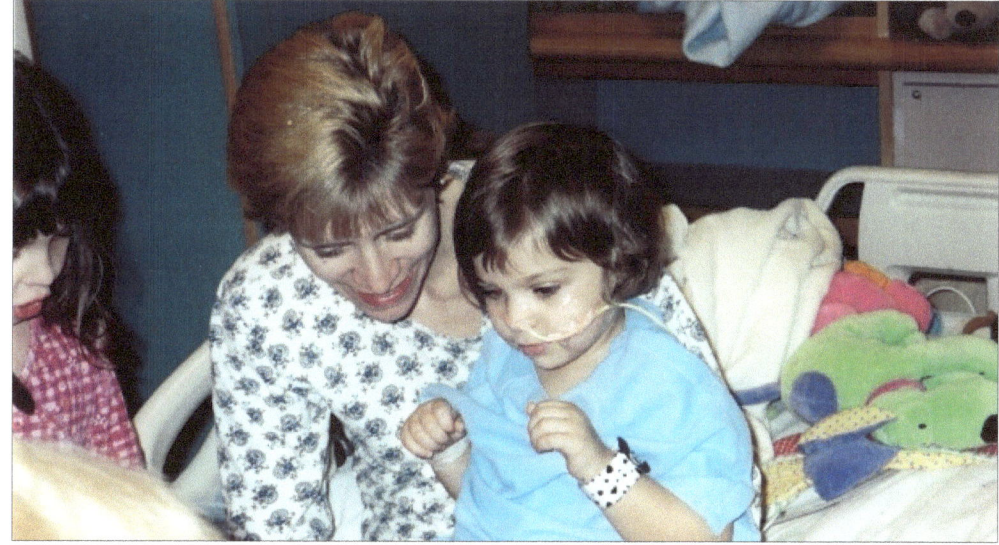

who was three years old, was diagnosed with strabismus, an eye condition commonly referred to as crossed eyes. However, in Olivia's case, her eyes went to the far corners instead of crossing in the center. I, too, was diagnosed with this condition at the same age and ended up having surgery to correct it. As silly as it seems now, I was devastated. I did not want my daughter to go through what I had. The doctor recommended patching her weaker eye in hopes that the other eye would become stronger and align itself.

When we arrived home that evening, I was met by Mike in the kitchen, which was really surprising since he normally didn't get home that early from work. I soon learned that the company he worked for had laid him off. I was shocked! I remember feeling like I had been punched in the gut, hard. We never saw it coming. His company hadn't given any indication that things were going south and, in fact, he had been given the opposite impression.

Mike began his job search immediately and was offered a part-time consulting opportunity following Thanksgiving, in New England, a short airplane ride from our home in Virginia. He left for the job the Sunday following Thanksgiving, and I held things down at home with the girls going about their routines as if there wasn't anything to worry about.

Two days later, on November 27, 2001, the girls and I needed to attend Hannah's Nutcracker rehearsal. She was so excited to finally get to do her part on stage and was bounding with energy. We got into the car and as I was pulling out of my driveway the girls were singing along to a Blues Clues CD that we had in the car. That is my last memory of the early evening.

The next thing I remember is hearing a paramedic trying to speak with me, as well as Hannah yelling, "MOMMY, WAKE UP! MOMMY, WAKE UP"! The paramedic asked whether anyone was seated in the back seat of my minivan and I understood why later.

I instinctively knew something was wrong with Olivia. My memory fades in and out, but I remember waking up in the emergency room on a gurney and Hannah sitting in a chair in the room. The nurse was telling me that they couldn't reach my husband on the work number I gave her but did leave a message on our home phone. I was so confused. I asked Hannah where her Daddy was and she reminded me that he was in New Hampshire. I apparently gave them his former employer's number and our home number which, thankfully, was transferred to the new house. I had also given the nurse the name and number of a close friend who was on her way to accompany Olivia to a trauma center.

Once I was cleared to leave the ER and Hannah had been taken care of, a friend drove me to the hospital where Olivia was being cared for. Ironically, Mike and I arrived at the same time. He had come home early from his trip, unbeknownst to me. We arrived in the Pediatric Intensive Care Unit immediately after Olivia had been brought up from the ER. The next morning, the Chief Neurosurgeon took us to a small, cold and dark room to inform us that Olivia had a severe Traumatic Brain Injury and a fractured skull. She was still unconscious and he did not know when or if she would wake up and what her prognosis was.

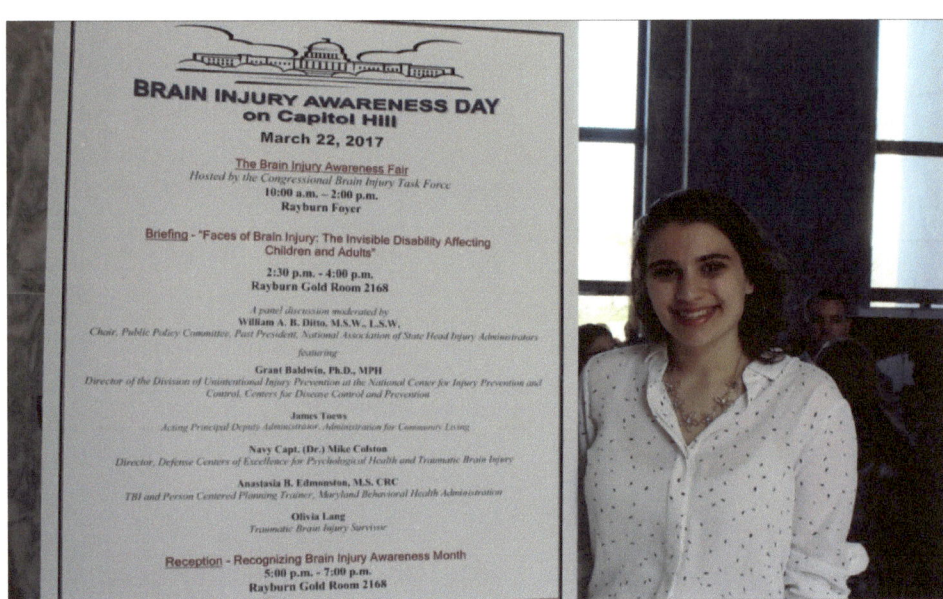

Mike told me that was the moment he stopped experiencing Joy. It wasn't a dramatic shift but one that continued to evolve over time. In fact, he hadn't realized how profound of a loss it had been until the birth of our third baby girl. He explained that he went into survival mode at the moment the doctor told us about Olivia's injuries. He turned his focus to getting his family better and providing for them and never realized that there had never been any deficit in his feelings. Of course, he experienced happy times during the six-and-a-half years between the accident and birth. But the happiness was just that: happy feelings. No profound joy. No jubilation.

I am brought back to the question of how I missed this. I didn't realize how much he had held back all those years. Our whole family had suffered terribly in our own ways, both physically and emotionally.

Meet Kelly Lang

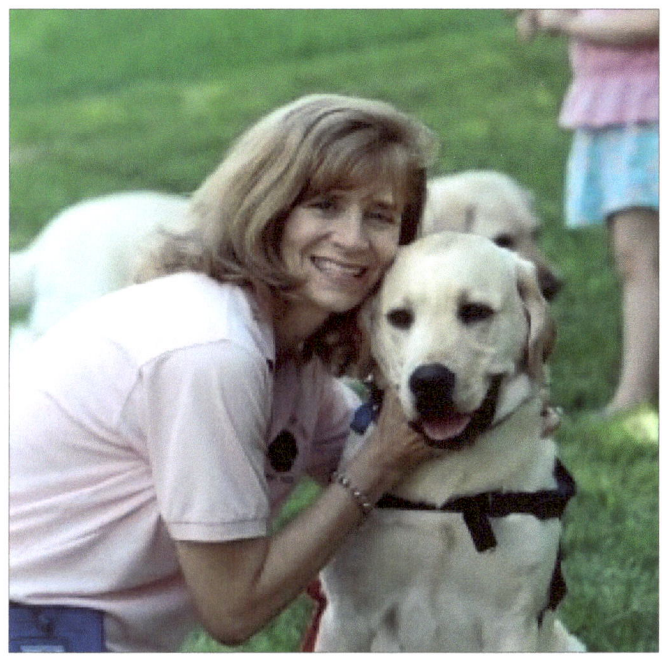

Kelly Lang, mother of 3 girls, wife, dog lover, TBI survivor and caregiver for over 15 years. Kelly serves on the Brain Injury Association of Virginia board, is a member of the Brain Injury Association of America's Brain Injury Council, and speaks with Brain Injury Service's Speaker's Bureau. She is also a Peer Visitor at a local hospital and is an inspiring author.

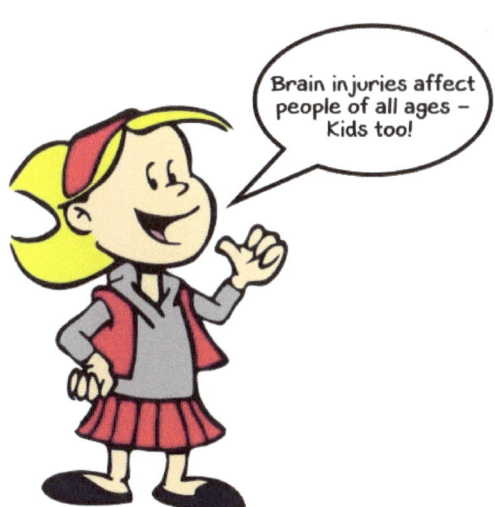

Brain injuries affect people of all ages – Kids too!

We all dealt with our pain in our own ways, and his way was to suffocate any feelings of joy until a renewal of sorts occurred. This renewal came in the form of this beautiful baby girl. She has made our family complete and has given her Daddy the best gift of all - his Joy!

The last six-and-a-half years have been tumultuous. We had to bring our daughter back to life. She needed to learn how to walk, talk, eat, and play all over again. She has also suffered from some serious cognitive deficits, processing issues, psychological effects as well as a host of other complications. We have never been told, "Your daughter will be ok." Instead, we had to continually hear, "We don't know what the prognosis is; every brain injury is different," or "The little girl you had before will not be the same girl who wakes up, if she wakes up. You will never know what her potential was because it's gone!"

Obviously, as parents, these words shook us to our core, but we had to remain strong and keep on fighting for Olivia to be the best she could be.

Our family now had this new bundle of joy who taught us so much in the few short weeks she had been alive. How much more would she be able to teach us? It is true that a birth is a time of renewal, a beginning, and something to cherish. Not only did this little baby bring new life into our family, but she also brought us something we didn't know was missing - JOY!

Brainy Word Search

Q K D T T J P Y Y G N L R
B G Y R S N E U R O N E X
V K J K P I J S I D C Y G
A B M T T D G T I O Y M Q
P Q R M Y M P O V S Y P N
H T L Z Y E U E L H O D Q
A W A A C T R I O O V N F
S L R R N Y I P N Y R F G
I Z E T X T E L T A U U O
A P T N H G E P I S R X E
D J A Y P E J R E B A C R
R M L V N R R L I L A Q K
G P M Y Q B D A D O N S Z
R G Y P M J R L P Y R Z I
K P M T L T R W B Y D M Y

Answers on page 18!

Find the Words!

Cranium
Anterior
Aphasia
Axon
Diffuse
Disability
Lateral

Neuron
Perception
Neurologist
Prognosis
Hope
Recovery
Therapy

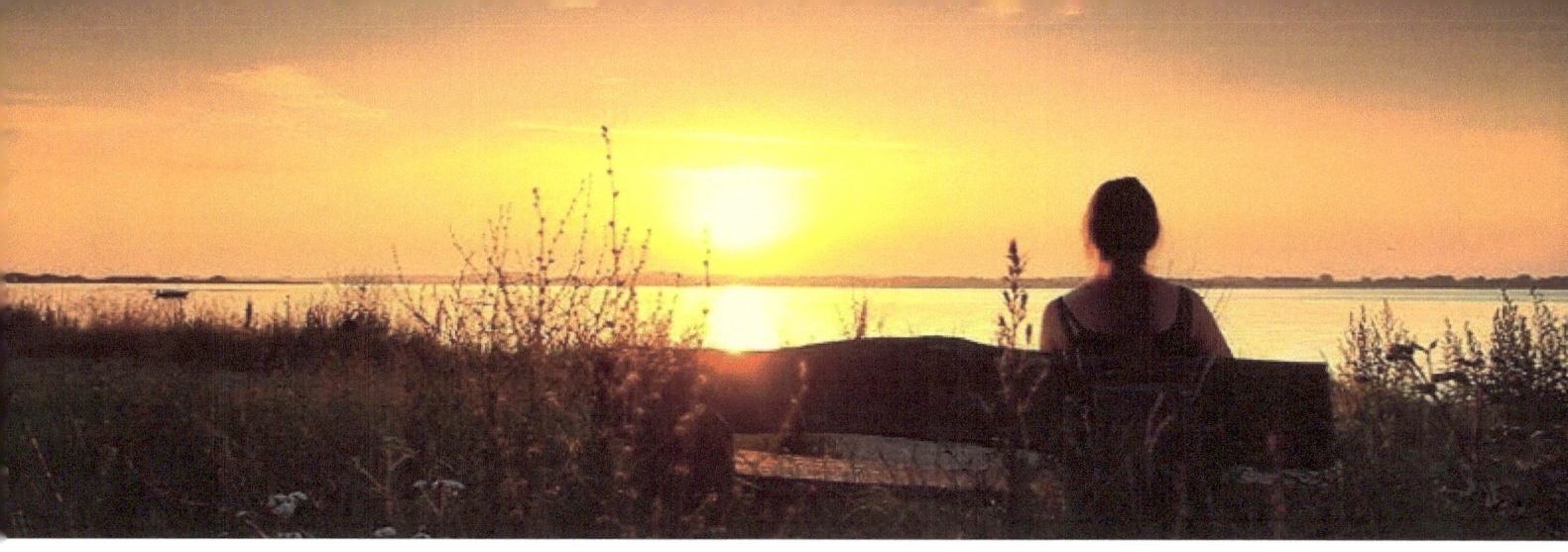

It's Okay to Not Be Okay

By Norma Myers

Recently, while going through my nightly routine, I was startled by the reflection in the mirror. Yes, it was my reflection, but not the carefree southern girl I used to recognize. I immediately started laughing and crying simultaneously. I laughed because my own reflection startled me, and cried because I didn't recognize myself. Sadly, my image could not be blamed on a mid-life crisis or hormones or failing to use anti-aging products. Any of these reasons would be a welcome culprit compared to the true robber of my identity.

Up until the night of the auto accident that caused the death of our son Aaron and left Steven with a TBI, both my husband and I held professional titles. Most importantly, we were honored to hold the most prestigious title of being Mom and Dad to Aaron and Steven.

A knock on our door with news of a car crash not only stripped me of my titles and identity, but it also left me with a broken heart. One-half of my heart left this earth with Aaron as he drew his last breath. Even while beating frantically out of rhythm, the other half kept beating with a purpose to lend strength to our son Steven as he lay in the ICU fighting for his next breath.

Four years later, as some of the dismal fog lifts, I can see that out of fear of letting anyone down, there have been many times that I'd proudly adorned the "*I'm fine*" mask. The mask is not healthy, and it can mislead family and friends into thinking that I'm the same person they knew before August 13, 2012. The truth is, there is no way to be the same Mom, wife, daughter, sister, aunt, friend or anything after every fiber of your being has suffered radical rewiring.

My mask is tattered and torn; it's long overdue for retirement. In retrospect, it was an unrealistic expectation I placed upon myself that I needed to be the same Norma I always was for the people in my life. I *wanted* to be the same. No mother willingly signs up to trade her normal life for a life of caregiving, TBI, advocacy for her son's needs, and being *that* Mom that no one knows what to say to because she lost her first born son.

The fear of letting others down is self-inflicted. I became so obsessed with ensuring that Steven's every need was met that I not only lost sight of myself, I lost sight of the fact that others need me too. They need me to say, "I'm not okay!" They need me to show up versus playing the "I'm too busy" caregiver card, when the truth is: yes, I am busy, but at times the avoidance game is more appealing than finding the strength to talk about my reality while everyone else is moving on with their lives. I know that my family, friends, and community will accept me for better or for worse; but I can't always accept myself!

If I were to attempt to describe all the ways double trauma has changed me, I would run out of blog space, so I will focus on one instrumental way my perception has changed.

My husband has lovingly adorned me with the title of being a "Noticer." Yes, even noticing and stopping to take a picture of a random, broken, upside down, but still standing headstone adorning none other than my last name. We stumbled on it, and it hit hard.

Ironic, I know! For some, this incident is too morbid to mention, but to me, all I could think was how many times I felt like this headstone inside. Broken over not seeing plans and dreams for me, my husband, and my sons come true.

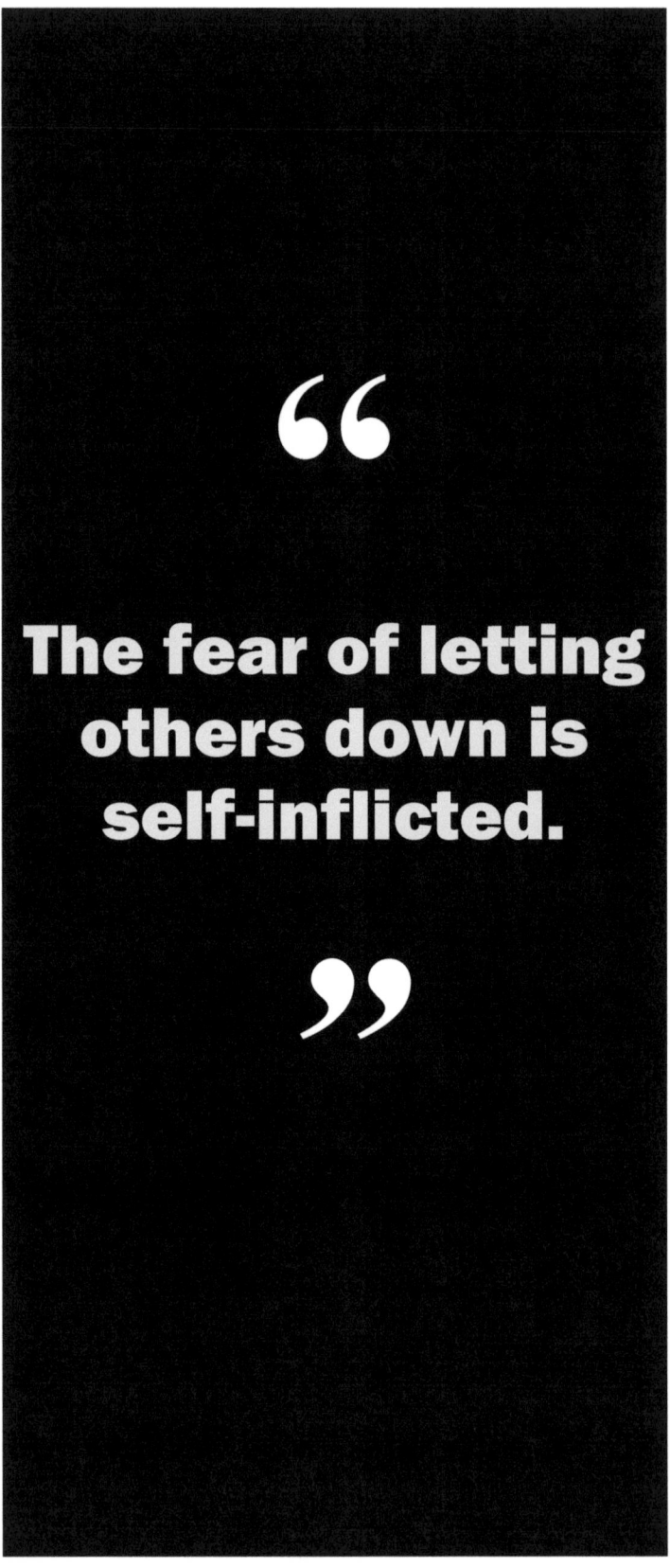

"The fear of letting others down is self-inflicted."

Meet Norma Myers

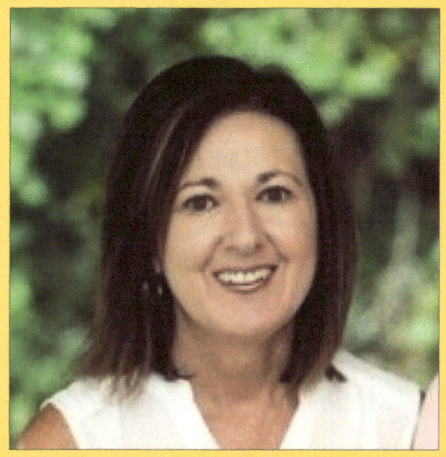

Norma and her husband Carlan spend much of their time supporting their son Steven as he continues on his road to recovery. Norma is an advocate for those recovering from traumatic brain injury.

Her written work has been featured on Brainline.org, a multi-media website that serves the brain injury community. Her family continues to heal.

Showing your emotions is a sign of strength.

~Brigitte Nicole

Upside down from the roller coaster ride of double grief; earthly separation from Aaron coupled with ambiguous loss. Still standing, but not steady. The headstone left me thinking about that old jingle: "*Weeble's Wobble, but they don't fall down.*" That's the Myers family!

Recently, someone shared these bold words with me: "***Do not miss those you have because of those you miss. Do not miss someone so much that you miss the people in front of you.***" Upon receipt, the words penetrated my heart in an unpleasant way. I felt angry.

Angry, because without intentionally doing so I know ***I have missed and have been missed.*** Raw tears are streaming as I type and feel those true but painful words. The heartache I feel from the earthly separation of Aaron is unbearable, but I know that he would not want me to miss our faithful family and friends who remain right in front of us.

It doesn't take away from how much I miss him; nothing could do that, but if I allow myself not to miss those in front of me I will gain a reservoir of strength to tap into when my own is depleted. Trust me when I say my genuine desire is to not only physically show up, but emotionally, genuinely and vulnerably show up—even when I don't feel like it! I'm thankful for those in my life who have not given up on me, even at times when I have given up on myself.

It's both frightening and freeing to be mask free. This journey is not for the faint of heart. TBI sucks for the survivor and the family. The loss of a child is not natural; it is unacceptable. I have learned many life lessons along our journey; some I prefer to embrace, and others I prefer to ignore. Above all, at this pivotal moment, I'm thankful for the healthy lessons that at first I ignored, but now I embrace. It's imperative to **let go of unrealistic, self-inflicted expectations, and** *it is okay to not be okay.* It's not a sign of weakness to admit this. In all actuality, I realize it's a sign of bravery to say, "Please be patient with me. I need you. I can't do this alone."

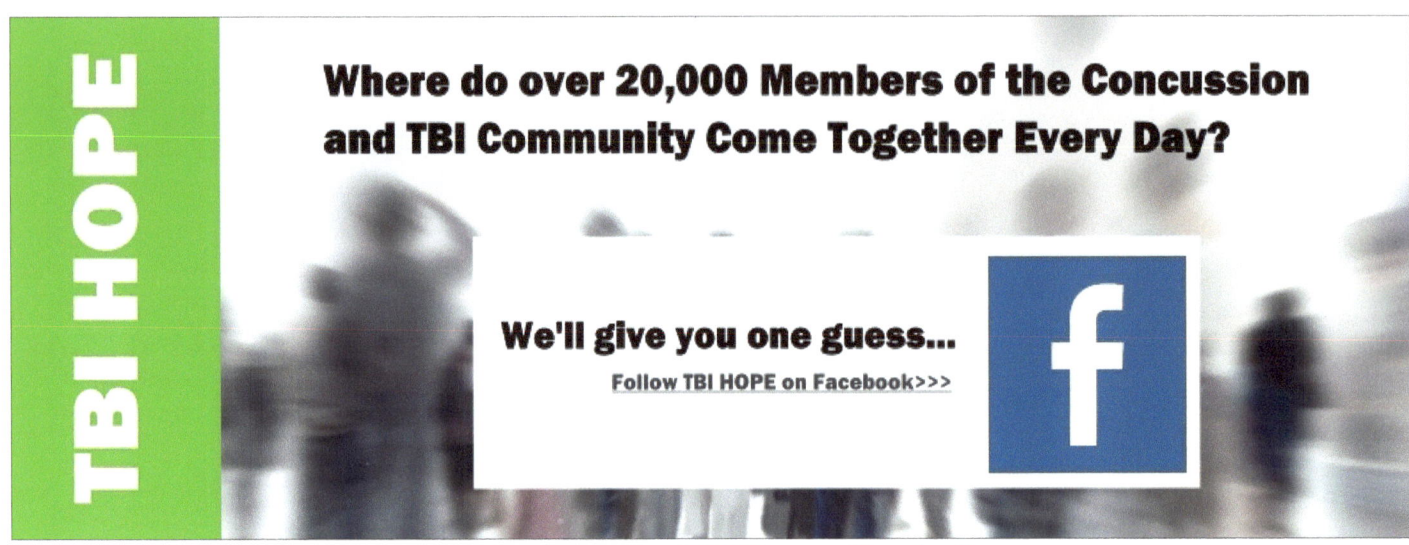

Brainy Word Search Solutions

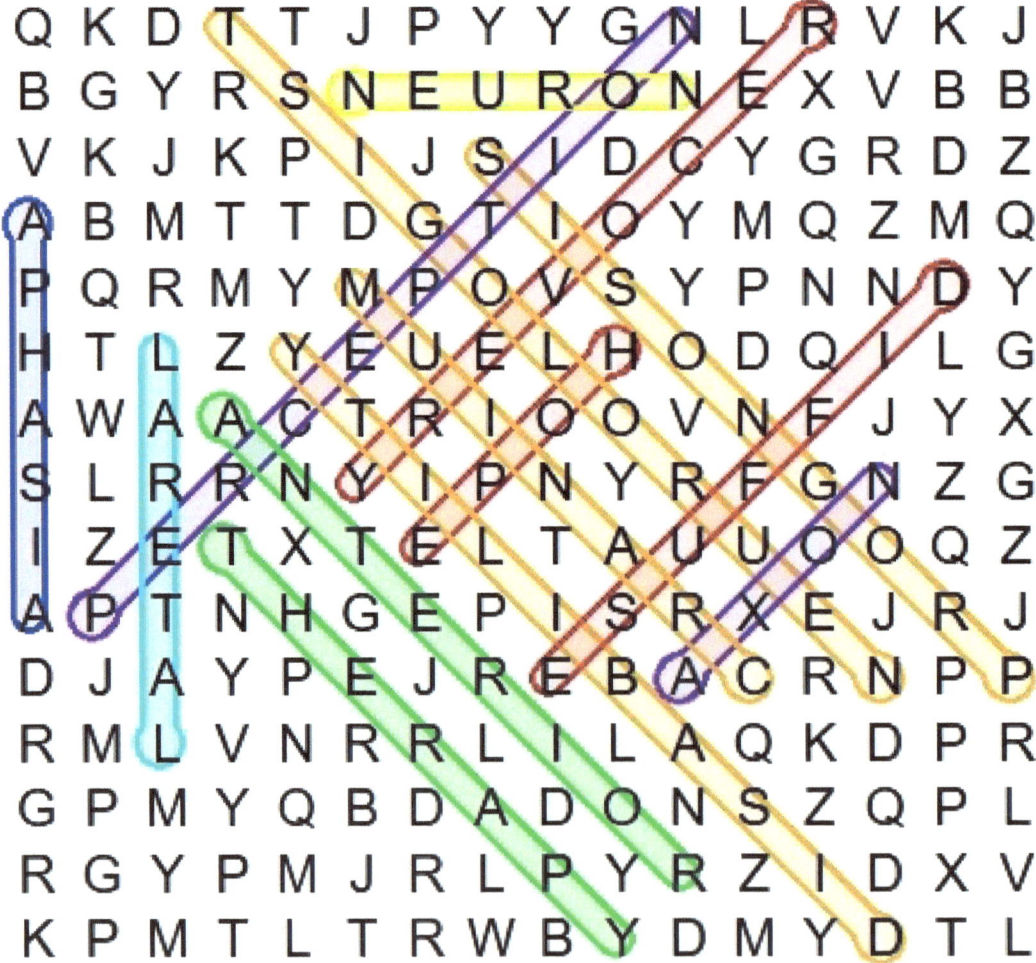

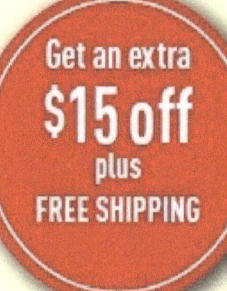
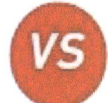
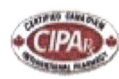 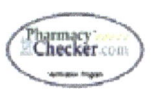 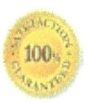 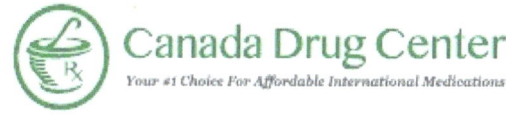

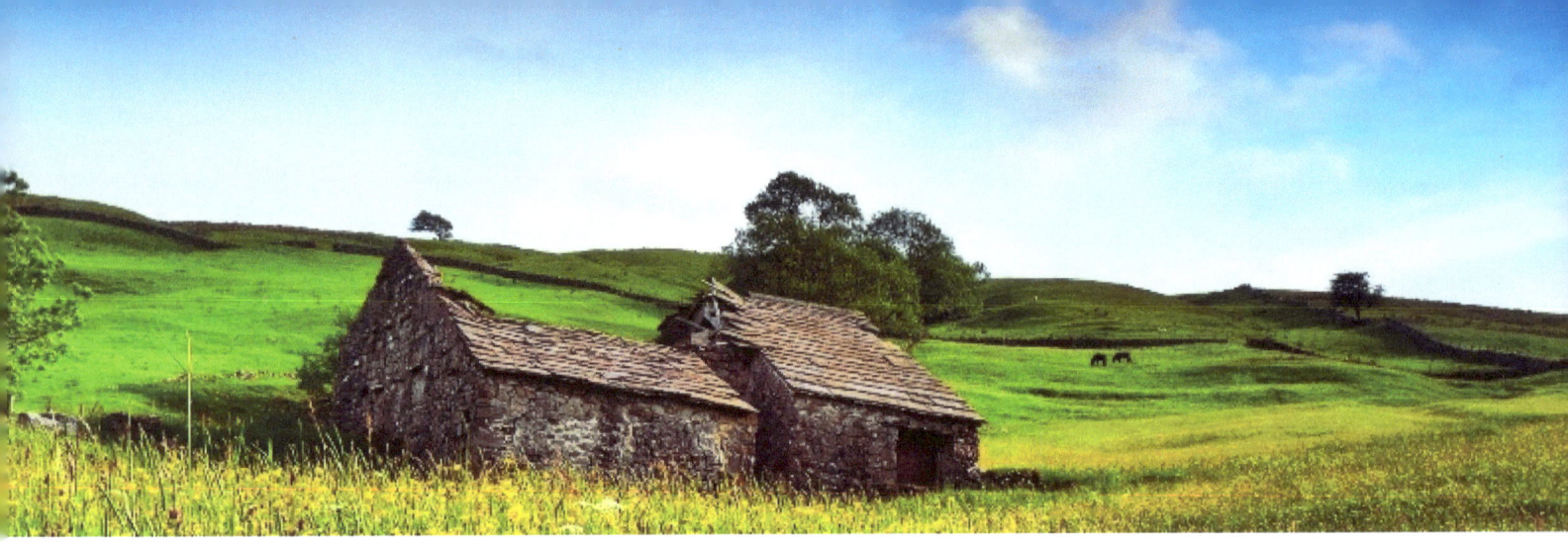

The Ultimate Goal

By Lisa Rainaud

Last week, my therapist Ellen asked me what my current goals were. My long-term goal is always to return to work to earn an income. I usually say, "That is the ultimate goal," but to be honest I am finding it is not the one that will bring me the most joy. It will certainly feel like the biggest success in terms of triumphing in the process of rehabilitation, but pure joy comes from the smaller successes-most of which have to do with my children and enjoying the simpler parts of daily life.

Today, the sound of a cow mooing was the loudest noise I heard for three hours. The wind was slight and the sun was warm on my bare arms. My children, ages 4 and 8, were alternating between holding my hands and running ahead to see what they would discover next on the dirt path. It was the week of April school vacation, I was almost three years post-injury, and we were spending the morning at Old Sturbridge Village, a living museum depicting life in New England in the 1830's.

That morning I had trouble eating. At first I was sent into thoughts of having the dreaded belly-bug that seemed to plague our friends and family this winter, but mercifully spared us. Then I recognized that this was actually an old familiar feeling, one that has been with me since I developed panic attacks post-injury. I was straight up nervous. I was taking my children on an extended outing ALONE - with no back up escape plan. "Fun day with mom," as we had been calling it, was not so fun for mom's nerves.

And if I didn't eat my waffle with peanut butter, almond milk, and pickle (need that salt for my low blood pressure) - I would be weak and lightheaded, lacking energy and feel about pass out - exactly what I feared. I forced the food down slowly over the next hour, taking bites in between getting the kids dressed and doing my hair. I WAS DOING THIS. Through sheer will or just plain stubbornness, I made it.

Walking down that dirt path, I stood tall and proud. I was feeling the small stones crunch beneath my feet and, taking a deep breath, I thought to myself, "*I am here*." I am here at Old Sturbridge Village, but

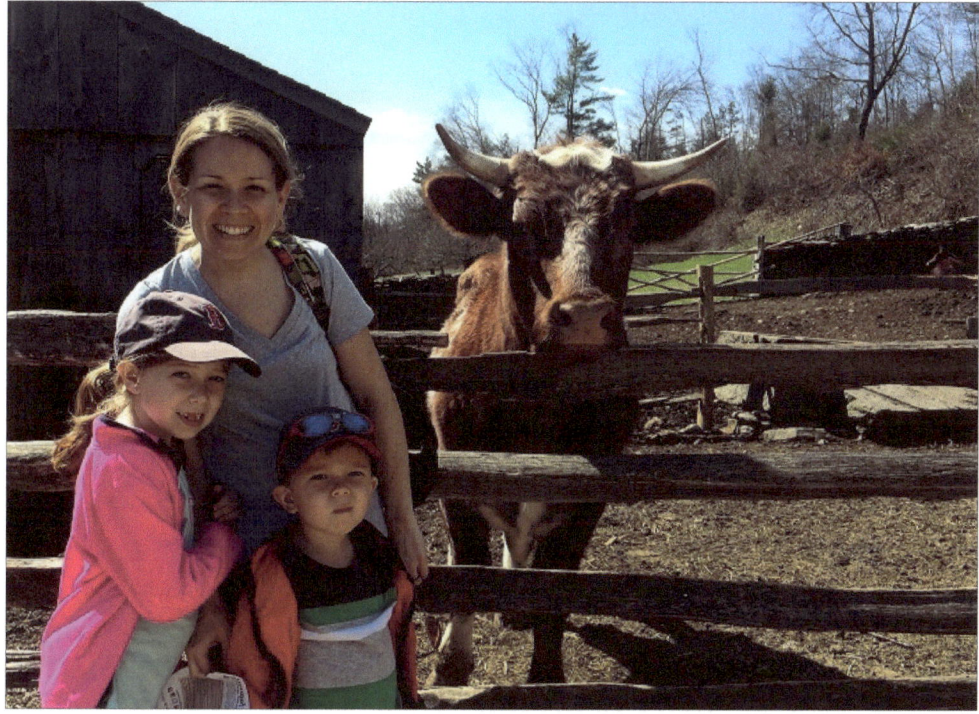

I am also here in my body, no longer a floating head. I am here with my children and I am so full of joy, because in this moment there is nowhere else I want to be.

This is my definition of joy - being so full of life and love in the present moment that you want for nothing and allow yourself to soak it all in.

I wonder, walking through OSV, why it feels like so much of a respite here, but it quickly comes to me as we stand in a kitchen and I ask my children to notice what is missing. No fridge! No microwave! No sink! All of these modern inventions that no doubt make my life more convenient also come with a price: humming, beeping, buzzing, swishing. It is not just the lack of cars and screens and electricity, but noise in general that I find so intoxicatingly peaceful.

As I write this, my children pull out their electronic keyboard with keys that meow, play music, and a background rhythm simultaneously. Why can it do all three at once?! It's maddening. In addition, I can hear my bathroom fan humming at the same time a dump truck drives down the length of the yard to our neighbor's house, growling, roaring, beeping as it backs up, finally slamming its dirt contents onto their driveway, metal door crashing back into place.

Down the street, a road construction crew has been jackhammering into boulders all day. The term "noise pollution" actually feels legitimate. But back at OSV, being inside a house is so similar to being outside in the woods. The lack of artificial noises makes me long for the quiet of a life in the 1830's. Would I even be considered disabled here? If I never had to look at a screen, drive a car, spend time in fluorescent lights or even read past a third grade level - might I be just fine? This thought makes my eyes well with tears. Maybe I am okay just the way I am. Maybe it is the world that cannot tolerate my simplicity.

So I rethink my current short-term goals. Do they serve me or do they serve the modern world?

- Tolerate more computer and TV time - especially reading on the computer
- Read for more than 20-30 minutes without fatigue or pain
- Not be exhausted by processing thoughts with background noise (ex. restaurants)
- Reduce/eliminate neck pain
- Be able to participate in cardio exercise - specifically that new beach body DVD I ordered that is still in the packaging
- Take my kids to the movies

Is it possible that the answer to my question is that they serve both, neither, or some complicated combination of the two? I am reminded of a quote by author Howard Thurman that I like to paraphrase: "Don't do what you think the world needs from you. Do what lights you up, because what the world actually needs is your light and the best version of you."

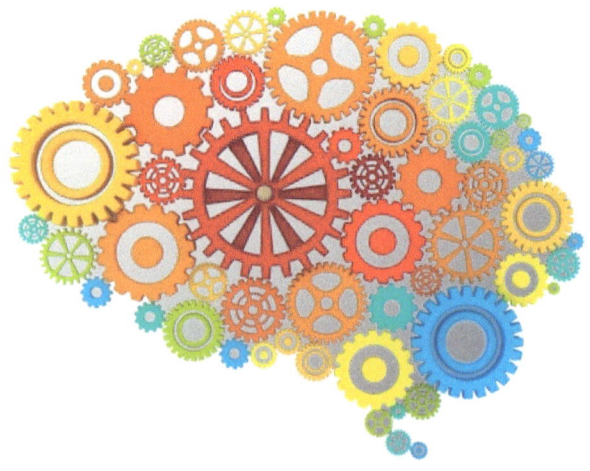

Meet Lisa Rainaud

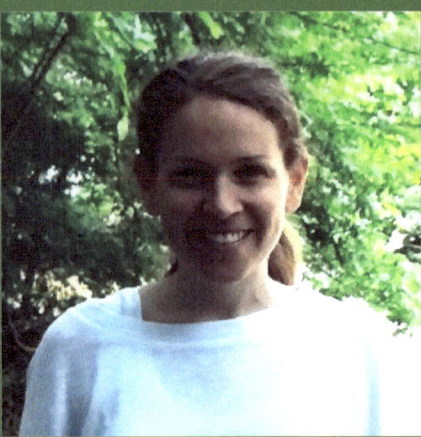

Lisa Rainaud is 36 years old and has been living with Post-Concussion Syndrome and Post-Traumatic Vision Syndrome for three years. An information seeker and therapy enthusiast, she is relentless in her pursuit of anything related to the brain that will help her better understand her injury and assist her in her rehabilitation.

She has found writing to be a creative outlet to deal with the emotional difficulties that come with a traumatic experience. In addition to writing, she enjoys listening to audio books, practicing yoga, walking, and spending time with her family and friends, especially in the outdoors!

Once a Type-A, always on the go personality, Lisa is being humbled by a slower pace and the practice of gratitude. She is learning that life's toughest experiences can be our greatest teachers if we allow ourselves to be open to the opportunity for growth through pain.

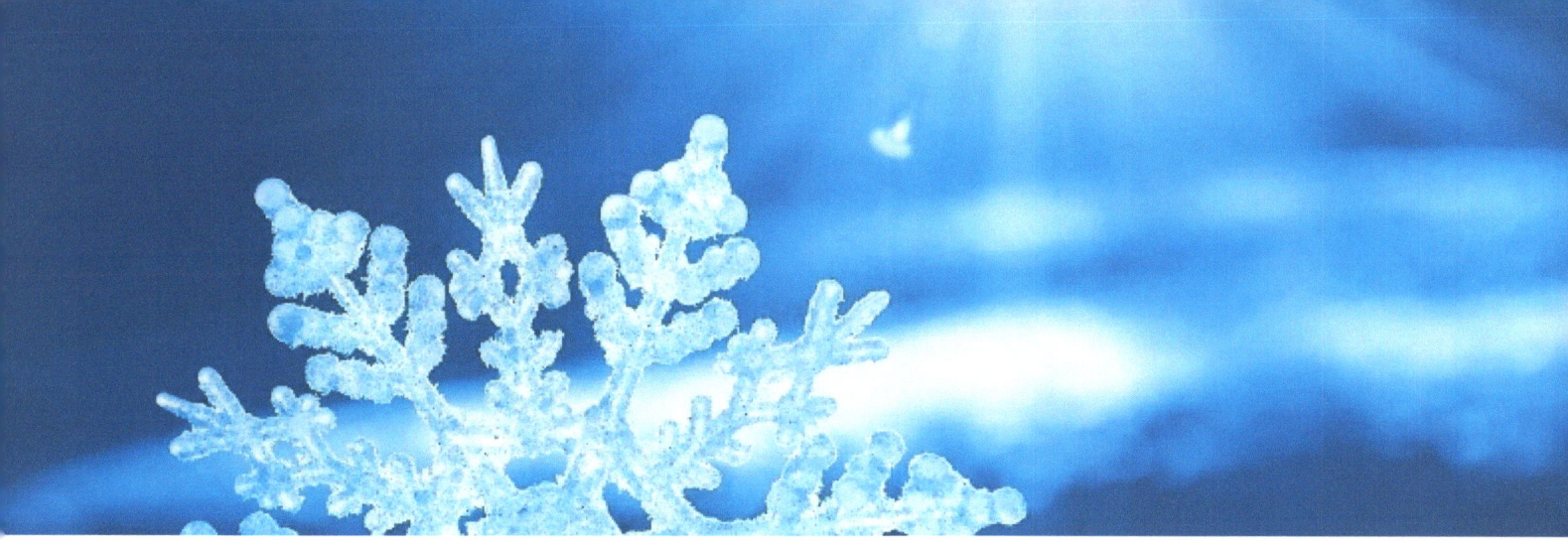

The Light at the End of the Tunnel
By Aislinn Fallon

Concussions are often compared to snowflakes due to the uniqueness in each and every case. However, concussions are not beautiful like snowflakes. They are in fact serious life-changing events people endure. Injuries to the brain are by far one of the most impenetrable injuries one can encounter. Brain injury causes neurological dysregulation; this means the brain cannot function properly. However, when one is concussed it is not comparable to having a broken arm. This is because brain injuries affect your whole body as opposed to being in one central location. Concussions cause physical, emotional, and thinking disruptions.

Concussions have been nicknamed The Silent Epidemic because they are not an injury that is visible to the naked eye. Although one's life may have been completely altered on the interior, on the exterior it will appear as though nothing has changed. Human brains are incredibly complex and have around 200 billion nerve cells and a trillion supporting cells. Veins, arteries, nerve fibers, a connective network, capillaries, hormones, and neurotransmitters make up the brain. It is no wonder that a single injury can alter one's life.

> "Concussions have been nicknamed The Silent Epidemic because they are not an injury that is visible to the naked eye."

Surprisingly, the location of the injury is much more crucial in the recovery process than one would expect. The right hemisphere of the brain controls the left side of the body. Meanwhile, the left side of the brain holds control over the right side of the body. This factor was significant in my own personal treatment. My injury was a result of a hard impact to the left side of my head, however, the left side of my body remained fine, while on the right side of my body I lost dexterity of my right hand in its entirety. It affected not only my physical mobility, but it also had an effect on emotional and many other types of functioning.

The right hemisphere controls creativity, processing facial expressions, and non-verbal communication. The left hemisphere is responsible for logical thinking, mathematics, verbal, and written expression. We can't leave out the frontal lobe near the forehead, which controls emotions, behaviors, social skills, judgment, and memory. There are many other areas of the brain such as the parietal lobe, angular gyrus, and occipital lobe, each with its own set of skills.

Concussions are typically due to a forceful impact to an area of the skull. The brain itself sits in a fluid called cerebrospinal fluid and, in fact, has very little internal structural support.

Due to the lack of support, an impact to the skull causes the brain to hit the skull resulting in what can be compared to a bruise on the brain.

Furthermore, you may get hit in one area but depending on the intensity of the impact, the brain could get knocked around and 'bruised' in multiple locations, making it harder to treat.

Although silent, concussions destroy a life in a moments' time. Concussion awareness is becoming more common, along with coaches who can now recognize the symptoms. With more awareness spreading, this silent epidemic is becoming less and less quiet. Concussions have the possibility to cause issues beyond when the brain is healed, but more often than not brain injuries heal in less than a year and life may resume as normal.

Some even heal within a matter of days. While in the moment, it might feel like the issues will last forever, but there is always hope and a light at the end of the tunnel. The more awareness about the severity of the effects a concussed patient endures, the better treatment one can receive. It's all about spreading awareness and making that light at the end of the tunnel brighter and brighter each day.

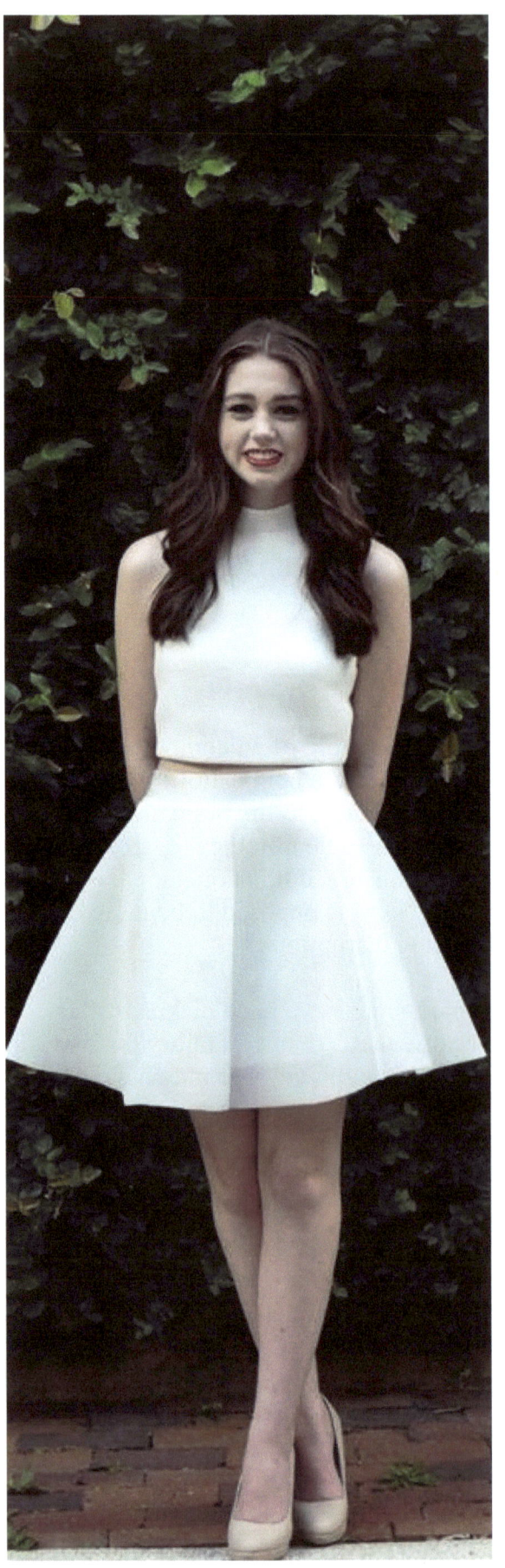

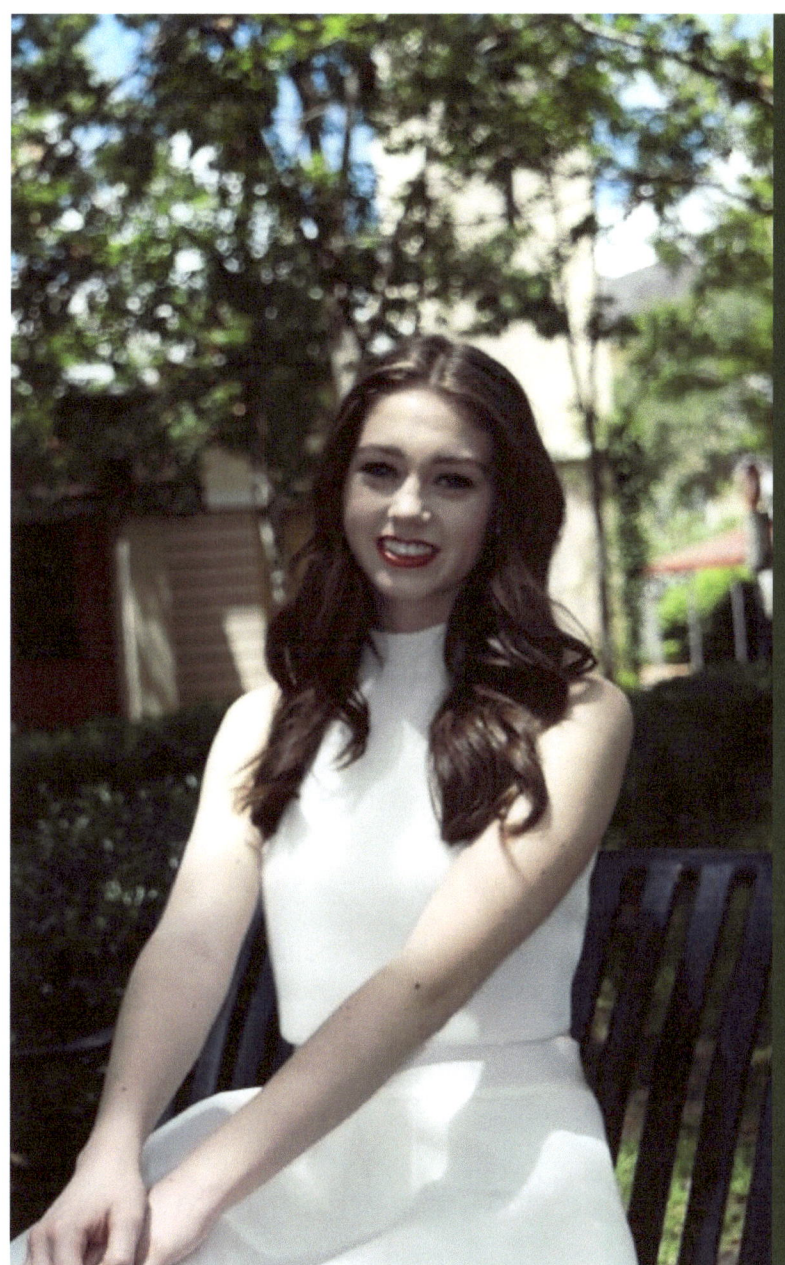

Meet Aislinn Fallon

At age 13 Aislinn Fallon had a concussion resulting in constant pain, inability to read, write, or speak properly, loss of dexterity in the right hand, frequent fainting spells, and many other challenges.

At 14 she had mostly recovered from her concussion but was diagnosed with four chronic illnesses as a result of her injury including chronic pain.

Age 15 she decided to create a blog to help those with chronic conditions live happier lives.

At 16 she turned that blog into an entire organization entitled 'chronicpain09'.

At 17 she became a four-time internationally published writer. Now at 18 she is taking the journalism world by storm. Her website has been viewed on every continent except Antarctica.

She is heading to her top choice college this summer with the hopes of becoming a pain specialist to help children live with conditions such as chronic pain.

Strength and growth come only through continuous effort and struggle.

~Napoleon Hill

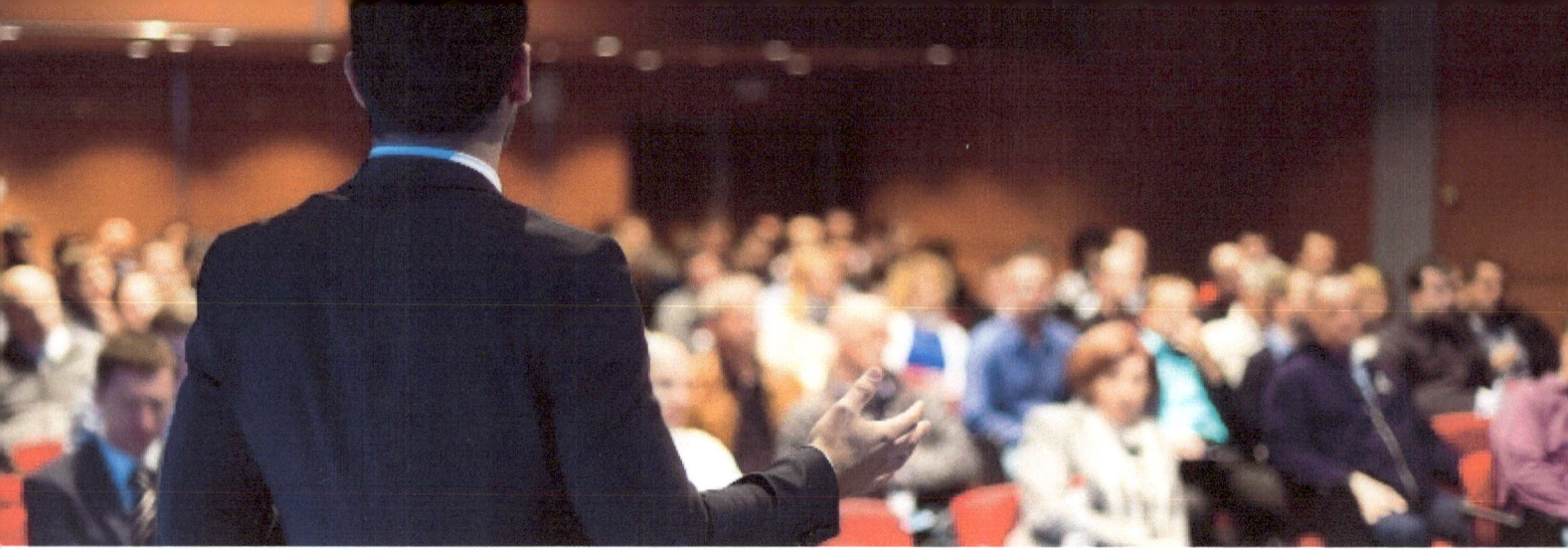

Return to Learn

By Amiee Duffy

I was fortunate to be able to attend the 36th Annual Brain Injury Conference in Massachusetts on March 30, 2017. What a positive experience! I would highly recommend survivors of TBI, as well as caregivers, attend. The experience of being in one place with so many others who "get it" was truly amazing and rejuvenating.

The day began on the highest note possible for me as the keynote speaker was Stacia Bissell, MEd, and Stacia's story is similar to my own in so many ways. As a fellow educator, I was nodding my head in agreement throughout her speech. I too told my doctor and employer that I would return to work after two weeks and was also shocked at the sensory overload I experienced after returning to teach, seven months later.

Two of the three sessions I attended were informative as well. I was able to gain quite a bit of useful knowledge in "Why Less is More: Cognitive and Executive Functioning Aids," and "Meditation and the Brain." Both of these sessions will not only continue to help me in my own recovery but will benefit the students in my classroom.

> "As an educator who suffered an mTBI and was able to return to work, I am in a unique position."

As I drove home from the conference, I had a renewed commitment to educating others on the effects of mTBI. So many people have little knowledge in this area. I am not only referring to lay people, but physicians, neuropsychologists, and educators as well. As an educator who suffered an mTBI and was able to return to work, I am in a unique position. I had a period in my life where I was able to learn quickly and focus effortlessly. Unfortunately, since my motor vehicle accident that is no longer the case.

I would love to have my old brain back. I would spoil her with encouragement and praise for all the hard work she did on a regular basis. However, even as every month or two seems to bring some

"I have been asked in a slow, loud voice with enunciated speech, 'Do you need help?' by a cashier at a supermarket."

improvement to my mTBI symptoms, I realize that my previous brain is gone for good. That does not mean that the experiences I have had with my new brain can't do some good.

I have had the experience of feeling stupid. I have been asked in a slow, loud voice with enunciated speech, "Do you need help?" by a cashier at a supermarket. And the answer to that humiliating question was, "Yes. I need help." At the time, I was confused about the process of getting my groceries from the shopping cart onto the counter in order to purchase them.

I have had the experience of returning to work and having colleagues and former friends talk about me behind my back, and even question me to my face, about whether I really needed that time "off" or make comments such as, "It must have been nice to have such a long vacation." Some of the time I would attempt to educate them, other times I would just sit back and marvel at how true it is that you can have decades of great work performance, but in the end, there are often people just waiting for you to slip up.

I have had the experience of sensory issues. I now know what my students experience when they are dealing with florescent lighting, the acoustics in loud cafeterias and gymnasiums, crowded hallways, and varying temperature changes from classroom to classroom.

I fully understand wanting to wear your hood up on your sweatshirt and to think it is not enjoyable to attend a band concert in the gym. I have had the experience of poor executive functioning and lack of focus and sustained attention. I have walked in circles in my kitchen and had no idea where to begin in order to cook my family's dinner. I have run the washing machine without clothes in it. I have cooked salad in the microwave. I have misplaced or "lost" items more often than I care to admit.

My job as an educator who has returned to work after sustaining an mTBI is to do good things with the knowledge I have gained through my experience. I already am more sensitive to the needs of individual learners in my classroom. I have taken classes and read books on trauma, sensory processing disorder, anxiety, and meditation in the classroom. I have no doubt that the strategies I am teaching my students will benefit them throughout their school careers.

The next challenge is to use my position as an educator who has returned to work to advocate for students who are Returning to Learn. There is much information on Return to Play, as there should be.

There really is not a set policy on students returning to learn in their classrooms. I believe that most educators have limited knowledge about what accommodations to make in their teaching practices and how to best accommodate students who are returning to school after a concussion.

I am looking forward to helping design and deliver professional development to educators on "return to learn" strategies after a student suffers a concussion.

Meet Amiee Duffy

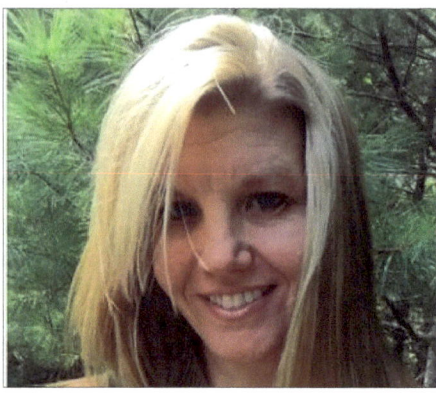

Amiee M. Duffy is the proud mother of three children. She has been teaching for over twenty years and is looking forward to using what she has learned about Executive Function and Working Memory in order to better serve all students in her classroom.

"Sometimes I have trouble getting my words out. That does not make what I have to say any less important."

~Brain Injury Survivor

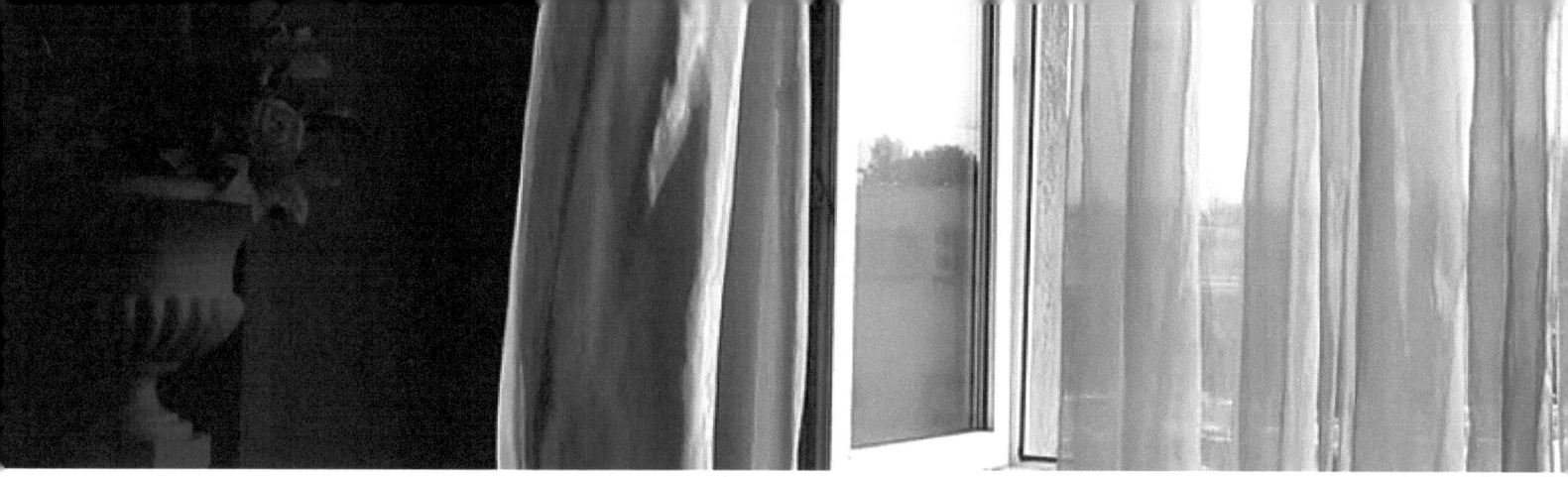

The Accident

By Jayden Pollock

Today, my motto is, "Never look back. Look forward," named after my brother.

Clean fresh air filled my lungs. We were at Swedish Hospital in Colorado seeing my brother the first time since the accident. I stopped abruptly and my grandma Jenny told me, "This is where he is." I took a deep breath and walked into the room. Grandma stayed behind to talk to one of the doctors.

My eyes were surveying the room like a hawk looking for its prey. "The Hero" is what my BFF Taryn called me since the day of the accident, for getting the neighbors to help my brother. Tons of flashbacks filled my mind. My eyes suddenly stopped on a boy that could not have been my brother. NO! My mind was screaming. Was he gone…..forever?

I heard the doctor and my mom talking. My mom knew I was here but wasn't paying attention to me. "He is not gone, but will have a brain injury. That window fall was two-and-a-half stories high. We'll have to keep him in a coma for two more weeks," the doctor told my mom over her sobs.

I walked over to my brother, ignoring the conversation next door. There was a big tube connected to his head. His eyes were closed, but not like he was asleep. I grabbed Colter's hand and I felt a squeeze, but not from me, from him.

My eyes widened. For a moment I wanted to jerk my hand away, my mind wanted me to, but my heart resisted me. "He does that only to his relatives," a familiar voice told me. I turned around urgently to see my mom red-eyed. She smiled and spoke again, "He'll be alright. It will just take time." There were many times I didn't cry, but now tears prickled down my face.

"I know it will be fine," I reassured her. My mom gave me a huge bear hug and we shared our sobs. Still to this day, I will always remember the past, but like I always say, never look back look forward.

Meet Jayden Pollock

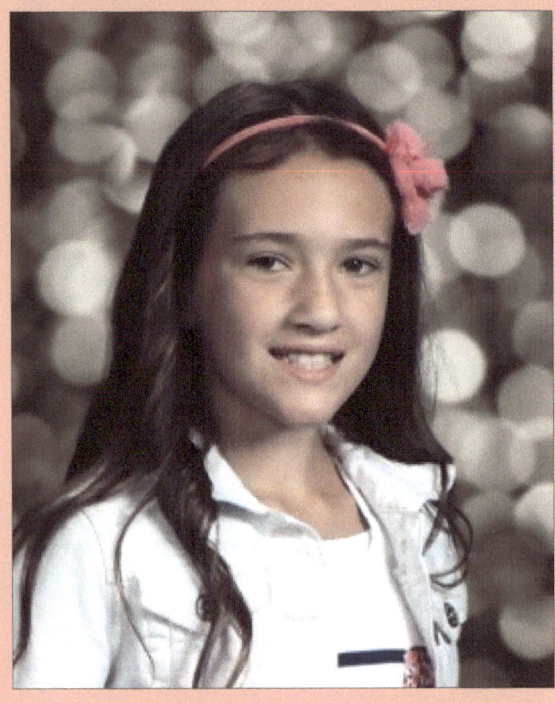

Jayden Pollock is an 11 year-old, 5th grade student at Douglas Upper Elementary School in Douglas, Wyoming. She is the older sister to her eight-year-old brother, a 2014 TBI Survivor.

Jayden witnessed Colter's accident when she herself was just 8 years old. She was honored for her heroic efforts and instincts in running to get help after her brother leaned on his second story window screen and fell onto the concrete below.

The local Sheriff's department commended her with their first ever Junior Citizen Award. Jayden loves writing and credits her success to her teachers. She wants to be a professional track athlete and a PE Teacher when she grows up. She loves to hang out with friends, play soccer & basketball, cross country/track, tubing, snowboarding, camping and playing games with family, and riding horses.

I Am...
By Jayden Pollock

I am athletic and proud
I wonder if we will win against K-Larks
I hear sounds of my brother hitting the ground
I see Taryn and I singing our favorite songs
I want the world to be made out of sugar
I am athletic and proud

I pretend I'm an Olympic gymnast
I feel my cat's fur brushing up against me
I touch an angel's wing
I worry I'll lose Autumn and Katie as friends
I cry when I get bullied

I understand why my dad shot Cookie-Dough
I say flying cars are our future
I dream for my brother to be normal again
I try to stop drama
I hope the universe doesn't become extinct
I am athletic and proud
I am Jayden

This poem was part of Jayden's Grade 4 poetry unit. For this particular writing piece, her teacher, Ms. Craig explained to the class to be raw with their emotions and feelings. This year was the beginning of Jayden's passion as writing has evolved into her favorite subject.

We've been reviewing publication submissions for a couple of years now. The courage expressed by all who have contributed to TBI HOPE Magazine over the year continues to amaze us. Moms, dads, husbands, wives – even older sisters have so much to share.

When we first read Jayden's story, it was difficult to not be profoundly affected by the courage of this young girl, her little brother now a brain injury survivor. If this story sounds a bit familiar, it should. A couple of months ago, we published Jayden's mother's story as seen through the eyes of a brain injury survivor's mom.

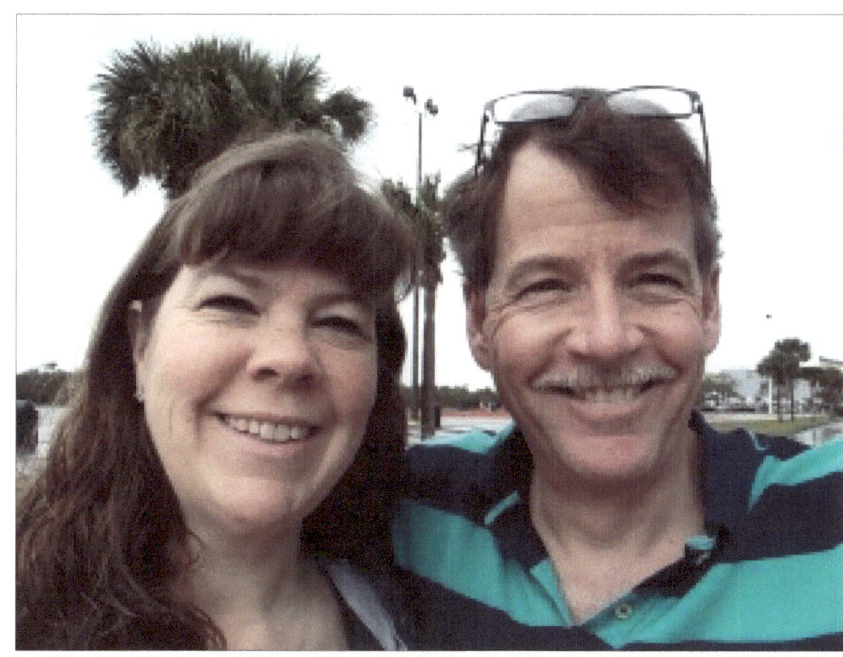

Brain injury is unlike most anything else as it affects entire families and communities. But one-by-one, as survivors and those who love them continue to share, the silence around brain injury slowly begins to end.

If you have a story to tell, and I'm sure you do, please feel free to reach out to us. Your story may be the key to unlocking the door of isolation to someone with a similar fate.

We've already got a full lineup for the July Issue of TBI HOPE Magazine. If you are part of an organization that serves those impacted by brain injury and would like information about offering printed copies of the magazine to those you serve, let us know. Qualifying organizations can receive up to 40% off the cover price.

To all our contributing writers, as well as our regular readers, a heartfelt thank you. TBI HOPE Magazine is now the fastest growing magazine worldwide serving the brain injury community.

Peace,

~David & Sarah Grant